RISKY BUSINESS

Disease Detective

Solving Deadly Mysteries

By

K E I T H   E L L I O T   G R E E N B E R G

Featuring photographs by
Leita Cowart

A   B L A C K B I R C H   P R E S S   B O O K

W O O D B R I D G E ,   C O N N E C T I C U T

Published by Blackbirch Press, Inc.
260 Amity Road
Woodbridge, CT 06525

web site: http://www.blackbirch.com
email: staff@blackbirch.com

©1998 Blackbirch Press, Inc.
First Edition

Photo Credits
Page 10: ©A.B. Dowsett/Science Photo Library
Pages 18 (inset), 19, 24-25: Wide World Photos

Library of Congress Cataloging-in-Publication Data

Greenberg, Keith Elliot.
    Disease detective / by Keith Elliot Greenberg.—1st ed.
        p.   cm. — (Risky business)
    Includes index.
    Summary: Profiles the training and work of a woman who has
helped the Center for Disease Control track down causes of vari-
ous deadly outbreaks of diseases, including the Ebola virus in
Africa.
    ISBN 1-56711-162-9 (lib. bdg.)
    1. Marshall, Katherine, Dr—Juvenile literature. 2.
Epidemologists—United States—Biography—Juvenile literature.
3. Virologists—United States—Biography—Juvenile literature.
[1. Epidemologists. 2. Marshall, Katherine, Dr. 3. Center for
Disease Control.] I. Title. II. Series: Risky business.
(Woodbridge, Conn.)
RA649.5.M37G74   1998
610'.92—dc21
    [B]   94-49616
                                                                              CIP
                                                                               AC

2

INTRODUCTION

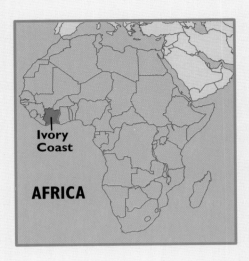

Ivory
Coast

AFRICA

In 1994, an African colony of chimpanzees suddenly and mysteriously died. They lived in Ivory Coast, a country located on the southern shoreline of western Africa. When three European researchers went into the jungle to study the deaths, one became seriously ill. Her symptoms led many to believe that she'd caught the dreaded Ebola virus from the chimpanzees.

Ebola had baffled doctors and scientists since it was first discovered in 1976. That year, two major outbreaks in the African nations of Zaire and Sudan brought the virus to the forefront of medical study.

At the Centers for Disease Control and Prevention—or CDC—in Atlanta, Georgia, the Ebola flare-up in Africa was being closely watched. The CDC was founded in 1946 and is dedicated to examining and fighting disease throughout the world.

Dr. Katherine Marshall is a "disease detective" for the CDC in Atlanta, Georgia.

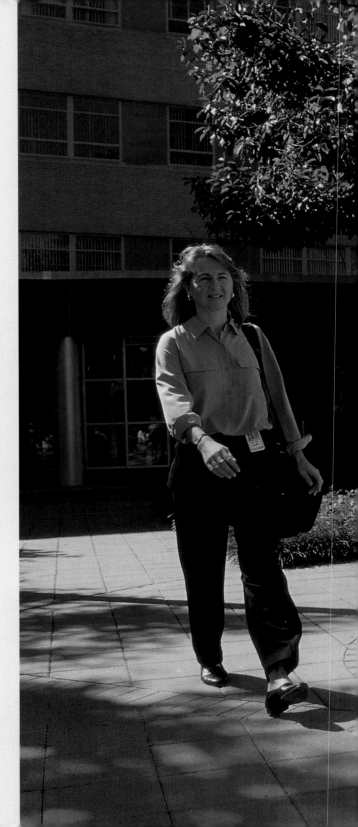

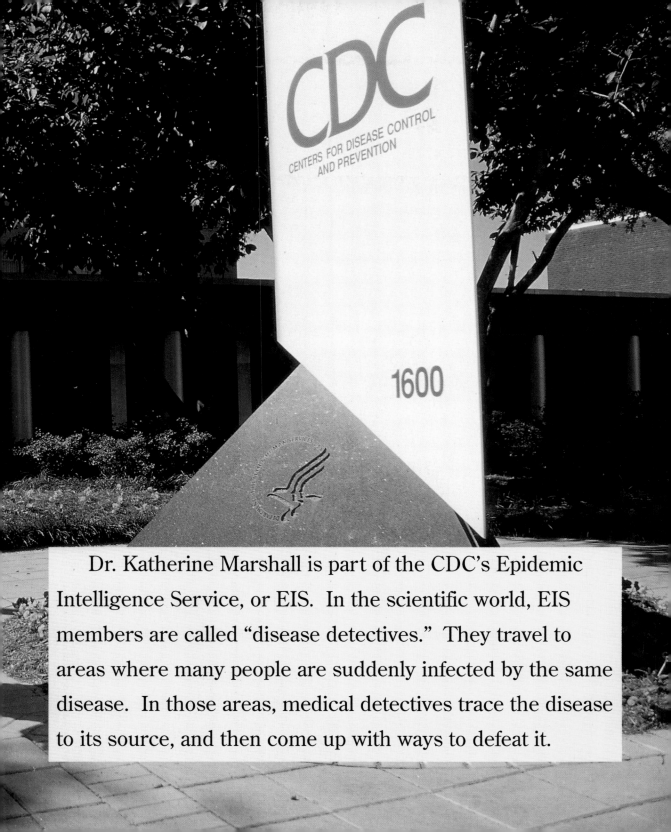

Dr. Katherine Marshall is part of the CDC's Epidemic Intelligence Service, or EIS. In the scientific world, EIS members are called "disease detectives." They travel to areas where many people are suddenly infected by the same disease. In those areas, medical detectives trace the disease to its source, and then come up with ways to defeat it.

As soon as Ebola was discovered in Kikwit, Zaire, the CDC's computer system sent the information to its employees. Katherine followed each development closely. The agency asked for volunteers to investigate the spread of the disease. Katherine offered to fly to Africa, even though she knew that other health care workers had died there.

"It seemed just too exciting to pass up," says Katherine, whose official title at the CDC is "preventive medicine resident." "The opportunity to study a disease about which very little is known comes along once every few decades. This was a chance to really use my skills."

Katherine can track the development of outbreaks around the world on her computer.

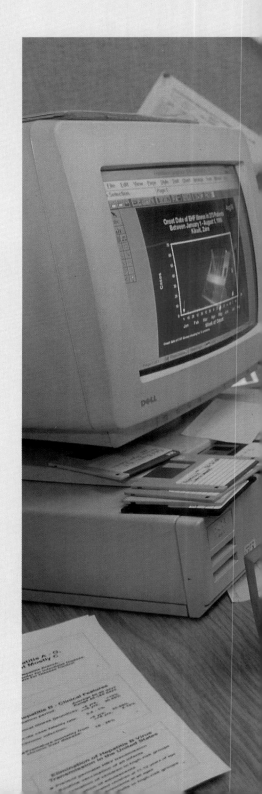

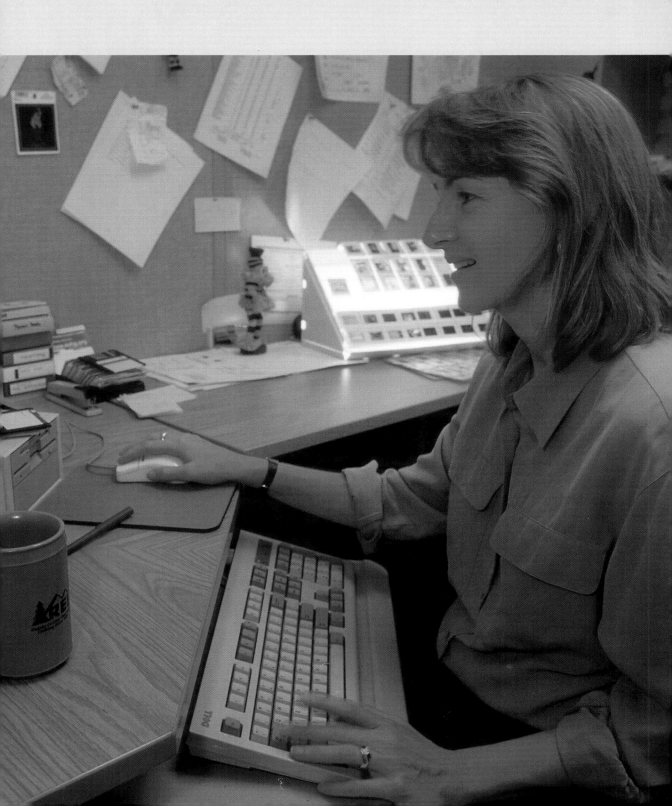

Katherine has always loved working with animals.

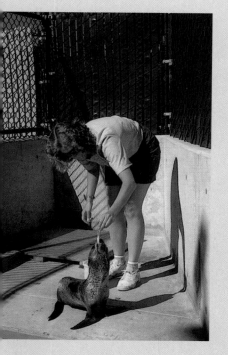

As a child, Katherine never imagined herself in Africa battling disease. All she knew was that she loved animals. During summer vacations, she visited relatives in Yorkshire, England. "They lived on a farm," she says. "I loved it there—the smell of the cows, the tractors, the fresh hay."

After high school, Katherine began studying zoology (the science of animals) at the University of California at Santa Barbara. During her spare time, she worked at an emergency veterinary clinic. She saved dogs and cats that had been hit by cars, burnt in fires, and poisoned by chemicals. "Cats love the taste of anti-freeze," Katherine points out. "When people change their anti-freeze, cats lick it off the sidewalk, and then get rushed to the clinic."

Katherine got her master's degree in public health from the London School of Hygiene and Tropical Medicine. Then she went to veterinary school at Colorado State University. As part of her studies, Katherine worked as an intern at San Diego's Sea World— examining penguins, dolphins and seals. She also worked for the CDC.

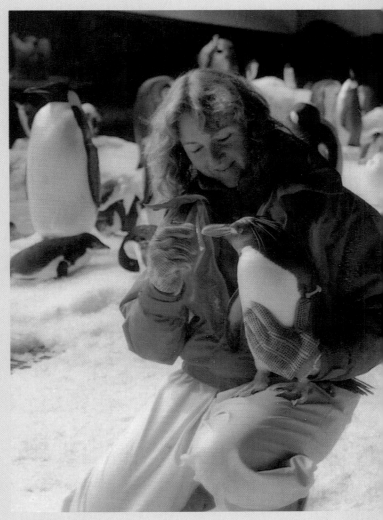

Early on in her education, Katherine worked at Sea World in San Diego, California.

9

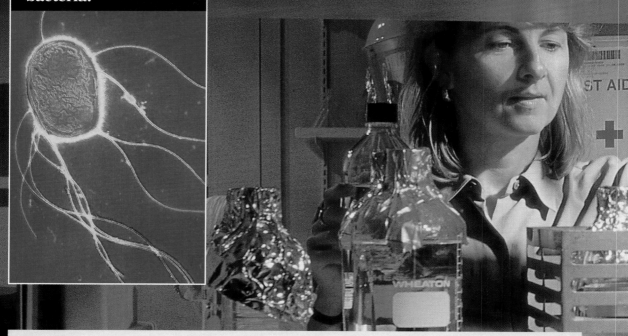

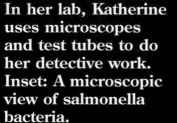

In her lab, Katherine uses microscopes and test tubes to do her detective work. Inset: A microscopic view of salmonella bacteria.

During her six-week assignment for the CDC Katherine was sent to South Carolina. Her office had been called because there was an unexplained outbreak of sickness. Many of the 800 attendees at a local convention had gotten severe nausea and diarrhea. The CDC determined that the problem was salmonella, a bacteria found in poultry and eggs.

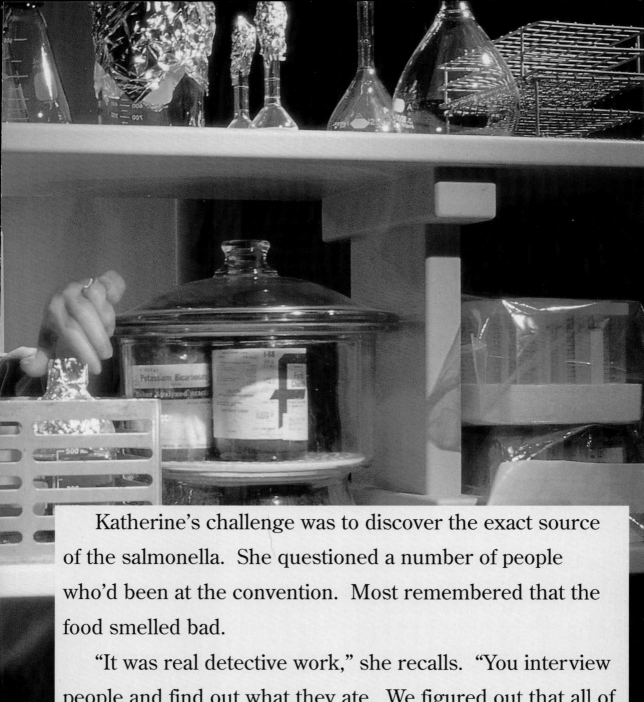

Katherine's challenge was to discover the exact source of the salmonella. She questioned a number of people who'd been at the convention. Most remembered that the food smelled bad.

"It was real detective work," she recalls. "You interview people and find out what they ate. We figured out that all of the sick people had eaten the turkey."

After some more detective work, CDC investigators got a phone call from someone who worked with the caterer. The person said the turkey had been transported in an unrefrigerated truck. The truck had also broken down on the way. The vehicle sat in the hot sun for hours before another truck came to pick up the meat. By the time the turkey was served, it had spoiled.

Katherine's time at the CDC sparked her interest in searching for the causes of disease. After working for the U.S. Department of Agriculture, she applied for a full-time job with the CDC. She was hired and assigned to the Epidemic Intelligence Service in Hawaii, where she had grown up.

CDC workers rely a great deal on computer technology to help them analyze their findings.

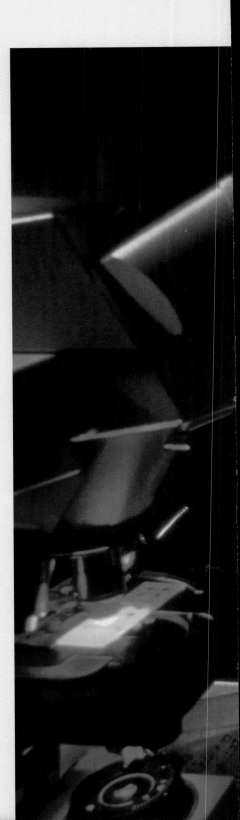

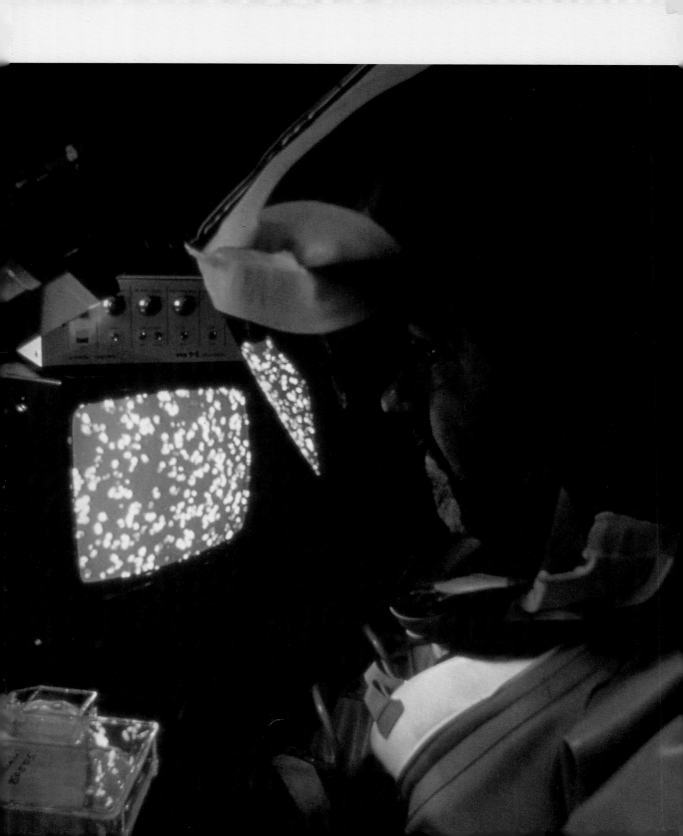

A CDC investigator tests some water for harmful bacteria.

Katherine's first job involved figuring out why a group of people got sick after a Fourth of July picnic. She learned that at the picnic people had eaten a Hawaiian dish called *ogo*—boiled sea-weed. "Everyone who ate the seaweed became sick, so we knew the seaweed was the problem," she remembers.

Researchers were able to get the left-over *ogo* for testing. First, they changed it into liquid form. Then they injected it into laboratory mice. When the mice died, they knew that there were toxins (poisons) in the seaweed.

When Katherine found out where the

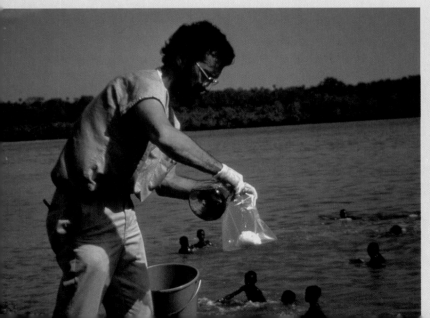

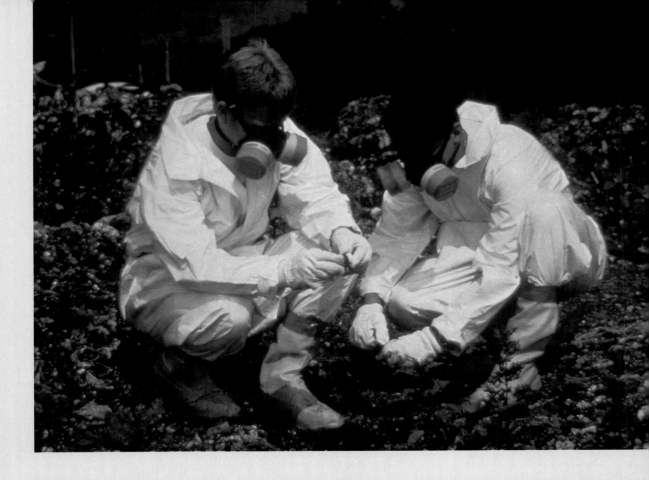

seaweed had been harvested, she and the other investigators went to that spot and began snorkeling. There, they finally found the source of the problem.

Blue-green algae was growing in a particular clump of seaweed. The algae was poisoning the seaweed.

Soil samples often provide evidence of environmental poisons.

15

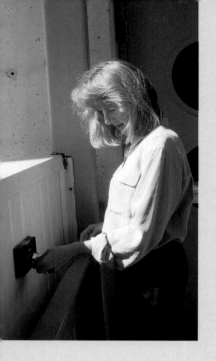

Katherine's 1994 trip to Zaire to battle the Ebola virus has been her greatest challenge to date. First, she flew from Hawaii to CDC headquarters in Atlanta for an update on the virus. Then, she and a group from EIS traveled to Africa, where others from the CDC were already investigating.

Ebola victims first experience headaches, weakness, sweating, and fever. As the days pass, fevers soar as high as 105 degrees Fahrenheit. By the

Above: Security cards are needed to enter the CDC labs. Below: Katherine prepares for a trip abroad.

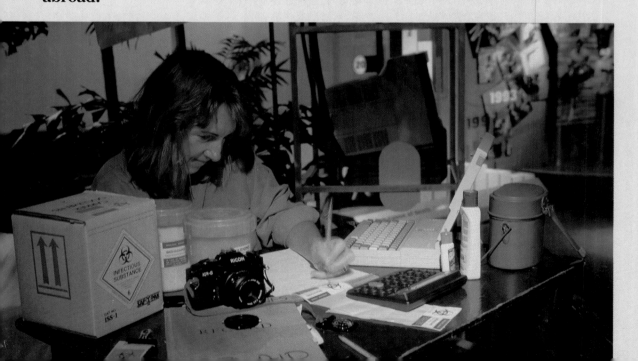

fourth day, patients often suffer from both internal and external bleeding. Blood oozes from the gums, skin, and eyes. The combination of bleeding and fluid loss results in death for 60 to 90 percent of those infected.

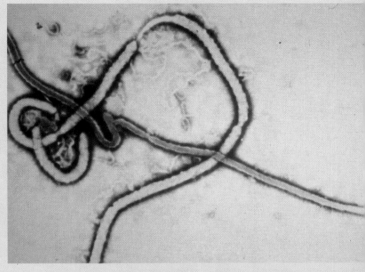

A microscopic view of the Ebola virus.

Ebola had remained largely undetected because it mostly affected people and animals living deep in the jungle. News of the virus didn't travel to areas where doctors could investigate the spreading disease.

A year after the chimpanzees died in Ivory Coast, a charcoal maker in Zaire fell ill. The man had walked through the jungle, day after day, cutting down trees. When he became sick, nobody knew why. Soon, he was dead—along with several family members who had cared for him.

17

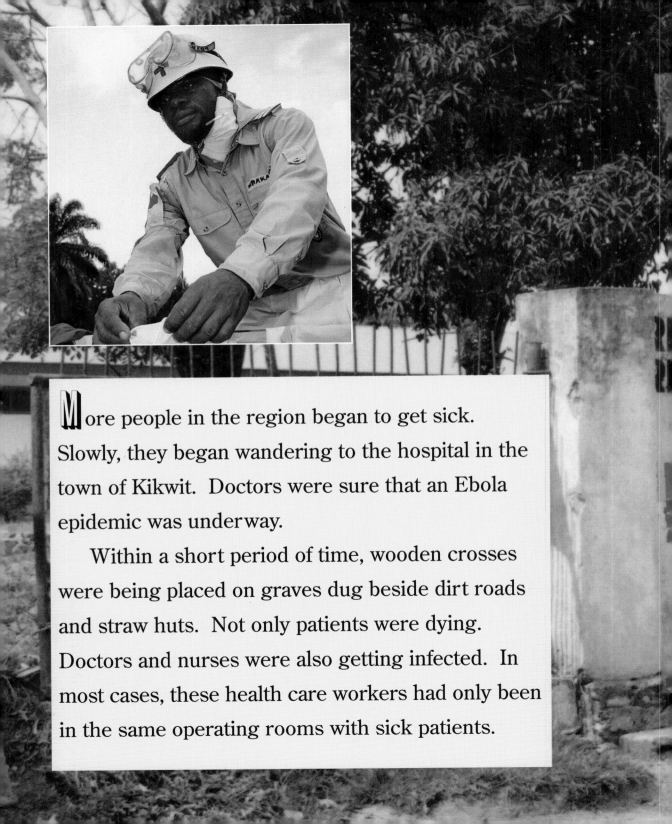

More people in the region began to get sick. Slowly, they began wandering to the hospital in the town of Kikwit. Doctors were sure that an Ebola epidemic was underway.

Within a short period of time, wooden crosses were being placed on graves dug beside dirt roads and straw huts. Not only patients were dying. Doctors and nurses were also getting infected. In most cases, these health care workers had only been in the same operating rooms with sick patients.

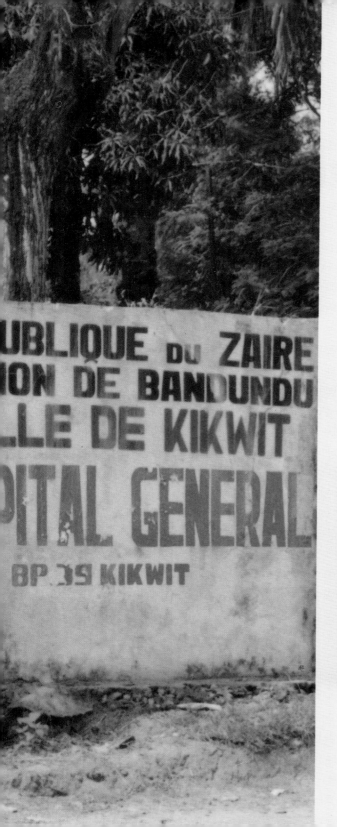

Katherine knew that doctors and family members who had contact with the Ebola sufferers had caught the disease. But a co-worker told her, "Don't worry. It's not as bad as it seems."

With so much death and suffering around her, his reassuring words weren't much comfort to Katherine.

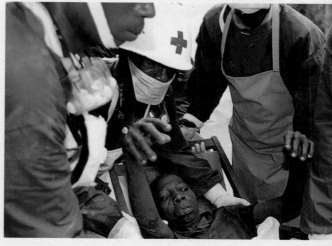

Above: Red Cross workers help to transport an Ebola victim.
Left: The hospital in Kikwit.
Inset: A Red Cross worker in Zaire helps to confine the outbreak.

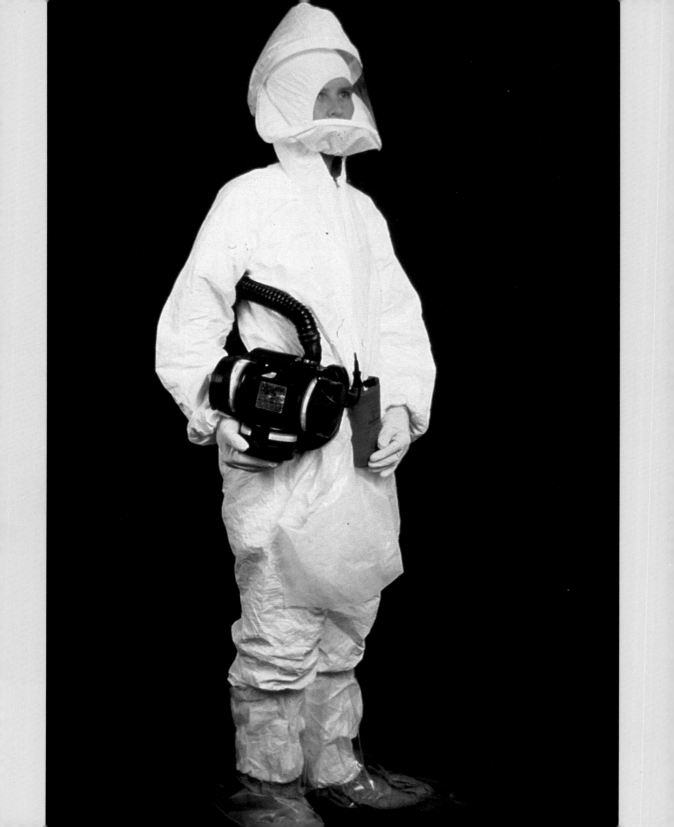

Within hours of landing in Zaire, Katherine was wearing a "bunny suit"—a hospital gown, gloves, rubber boots, and mask. Right away she began taking tissue samples from some of the people who had recently died of Ebola. Because it is so dangerous, scientists always wear protective clothing when working with the virus.

At the CDC's office in Atlanta, the dangerous samples are inspected in a special lab. This lab is called a Biosafety Level Four laboratory. It has its own air, water, and waste removal systems.

In dangerous situations, CDC workers wear special protective clothing, often called "bunny suits."

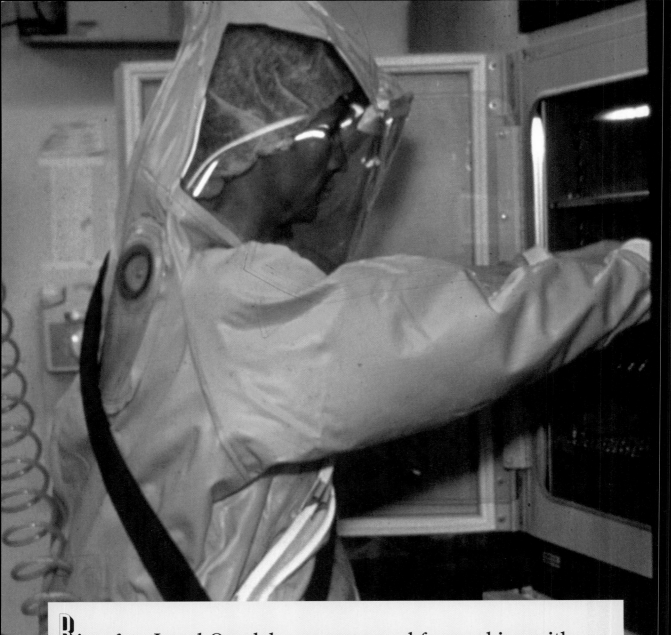

Biosafety Level One labs are reserved for working with organisms that do not cause disease in humans. Biosafety Level Two labs are for viruses—like Hepatitis B—that carry a slight risk. Biosafety Level Three labs are for diseases

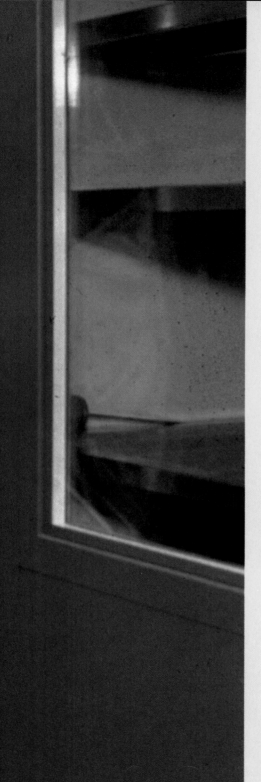

that are carried through the air, like tuberculosis. Observations are made in unique "biological safety cabinets," which are cut off from all outside air. Biosafety Level Four is the top level. It is restricted to the world's most dangerous and deadly diseases.

The purpose of the CDC's biosafety unit is to guarantee that "the bugs stay in the labs where they belong and don't walk out with the scientists," says CDC's Henry Mathews, who oversees the labs.

Workers in the CDC's Biosafety labs must take many precautions to be safe.

23

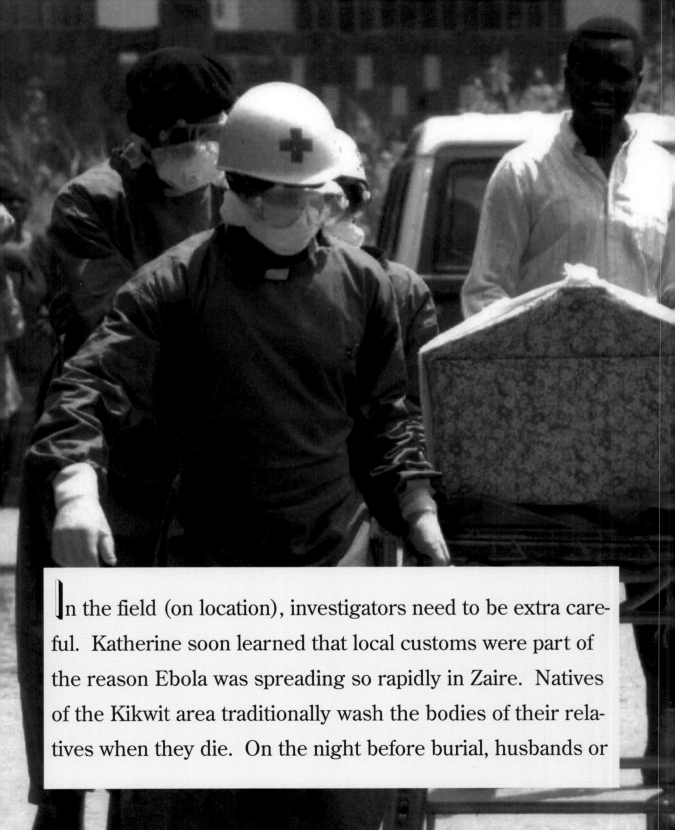

In the field (on location), investigators need to be extra careful. Katherine soon learned that local customs were part of the reason Ebola was spreading so rapidly in Zaire. Natives of the Kikwit area traditionally wash the bodies of their relatives when they die. On the night before burial, husbands or

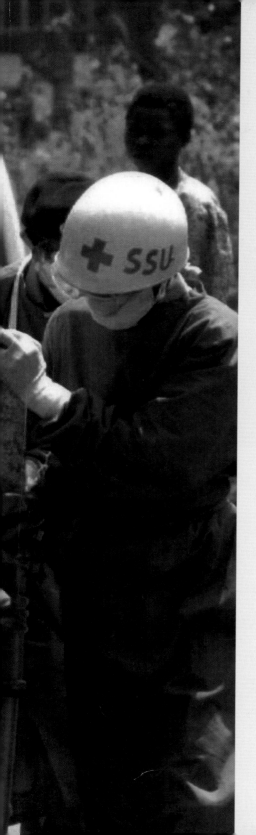

wives will sleep in the same bed as their dead spouses—as a way of saying goodbye. These customs were allowing the germs to spread rapidly. To slow the spread of the disease, the Red Cross collected the bodies of people as soon as they died.

Investigators determined that the easiest way to stop Ebola was to track down the "reservoir," or source of the illness. The reservoir is "an animal that carries the virus, but doesn't get sick from it," Katherine explains. "You have to understand that the virus must live somewhere before it emerges and begins infecting people."

Red Cross workers in Zaire needed to control what happened to the bodies of those who died from Ebola.

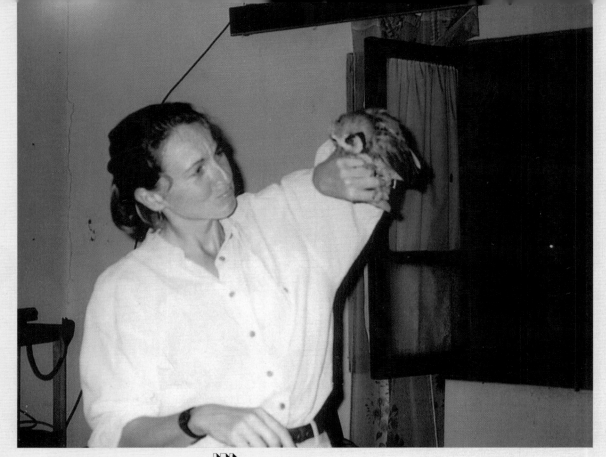

An owl named "Ebola" made friends with local CDC workers in Kikwit.

Workers for the CDC put out the word that they wanted to examine every breed of animal in the region. At the house where Katherine and the other inspectors were staying, people arrived continually with different types of animals: tree snakes, monkeys, exotic birds, even giant rats.

In Kikwit, the hospital staff eventually stopped getting infected with the virus. "We simply told the doctors and nurses to wear gloves, masks, and gowns," Katherine explains.

This tiger was tested to see if it was an Ebola carrier.

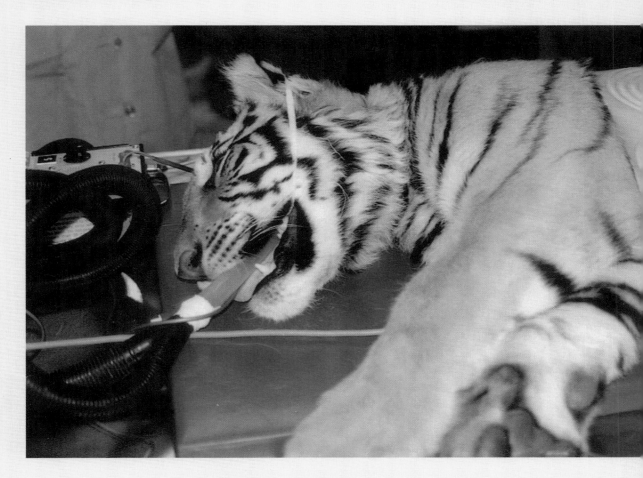

People from the CDC, along with members of other organizations, went into villages and educated people about Ebola. The main message: Bring your sick to the hospital immediately.

Within four months of the CDC's arrival in Kikwit, the spread of Ebola in the area was stopped. But there have been other outbreaks. In May 1996, a group of 13 people died after eating a chimpanzee in the nation of Gabon. Five months later, 8 more people died in the same region. The reservoir of the disease has yet to be located. "We're still looking," Katherine says.

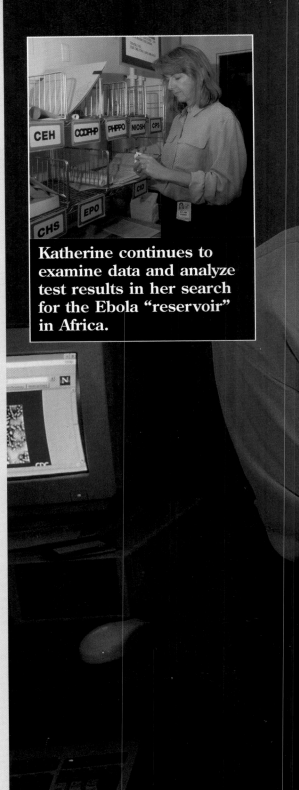

Katherine continues to examine data and analyze test results in her search for the Ebola "reservoir" in Africa.

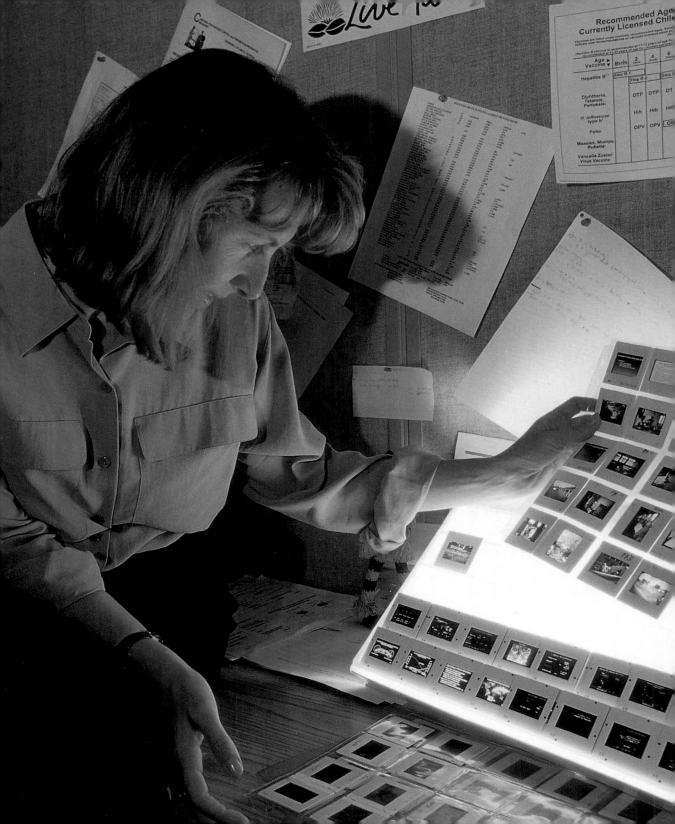

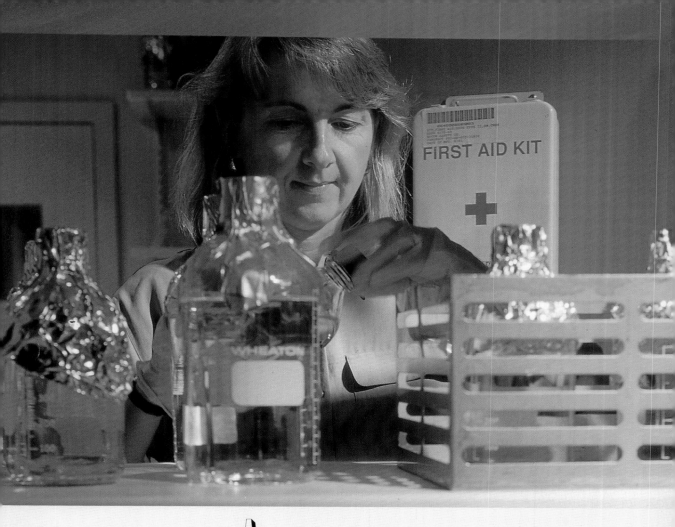

Searching for answers to disease outbreaks can often take months, even years.

After her visit to Zaire, Katherine took a year-long assignment at CDC headquarters in Atlanta. She now lives in San Francisco with her husband, Paul Hofmann, an engineer.

No matter where her career as a disease detective takes her next, the people of Kikwit will always hold a special place in Katherine's heart. "They were great," she says, "hard-working, friendly, appreciative of all we were trying to do. This was the kind of experience I always wanted to have."

Katherine poses for a photo with many of the friends she made in Kikwit.

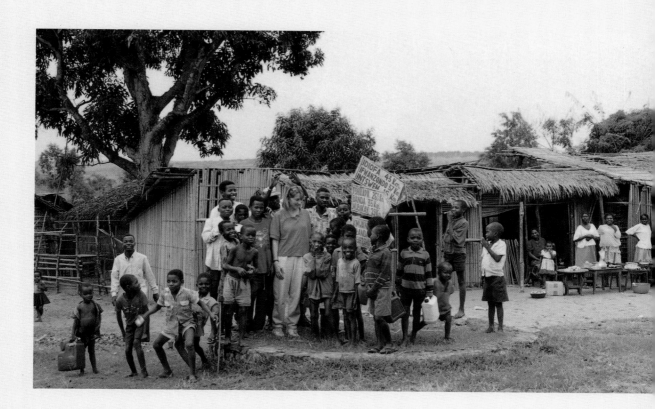

FOR MORE INFORMATION

Books:

Graham, Ian. *Fighting Disease.* Chatham, NJ: Raintree Steck-Vaughn, 1995.

Lampton, Christopher. *Epidemic.* Brookfield, CT: Millbrook Press, 1992.

Reid, S. and P. Fara, *Scientists.* Newton, MA: Educational Development Center, 1993.

Web Sites:

http://www.comet.chv.va.us/quill

An in-depth look at a variety of different cells and how they function. Videos include the tracking of an HIV infection through a lymphocyte and the making of antibodies.

http://whyfiles.news.wisc.edu

Articles on the scientific "wheres, whys, and hows" behind today's headlines.

http://commtechlab.msu.edu/CTLProjects/dlc-me

Interesting graphics and information, including a "Microbe Zoo" with pictures and data about unique microbes.

http://www.cdc.gov

CDC's homepage; information about the CDC, diseases and bacteria; helpful notices for travelers.

INDEX